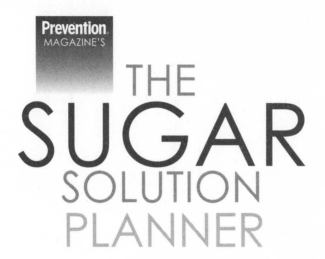

Prevention MAGAZINE'S
THE SUGAR SOLUTION PLANNER

Prevention. MAGAZINE'S

THE
SUGAR
SOLUTION
PLANNER

Track your progress toward

optimal blood sugar control

Sarí Harrar and the Editors of **Prevention.** magazine

RODALE

Cover photograph recipe is Ginger Frozen Yogurt with Sweet Plum Sauce from the companion book, *Prevention Magazine's The Sugar Solution Quick & Easy Recipes,* page 181.

Book design by Christina Gaugler

Library of Congress Cataloging-in-Publication Data

Harrar, Sarí.
   Prevention magazine's the sugar solution planner : track your progress toward optimal blood sugar control / Sarí Harrar and the editors of Prevention magazine.
      p.   cm.
   ISBN-13 978–1–59486–619–7 paperback
   ISBN-10 1–59486–619–8 paperback
   1. Blood sugar—Popular works. 2. Nutrition—Popular works.   I. Prevention Magazine Health Books. II. Title.   III. Title: Sugar solution planner track your progress toward optimal blood sugar control.
QP99.3.B5H37 2006
612.1'2—dc22   2006012628

2 4 6 8 10 9 7 5 3 1   paperback

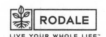

CONTENTS

INTRODUCTION

The *Sugar Solution* program can help you bring your lifestyle back into harmony with your body's true needs. It's a simple, delicious, healthy approach that reduces your blood sugar and dampens elevated levels of insulin, a key hormone for blood sugar control. The advantage: You can step off the sugar "spike and dip" roller coaster that contributes to stubborn weight gain, fatigue, moodiness, and cravings. You'll protect yourself against the profoundly damaging effects of high insulin and high blood sugar. You'll feel more energetic. (If you have diabetes, don't stop using your medication: This program can work with your doctor's treatment plan to help keep your blood sugar levels lower and steadier.) The details:

STRATEGY #1: EAT SMART

The *Sugar Solution* eating plan can help you lose weight now, keep it off forever, and protect you from a wide array of serious health problems, from heart attack and stroke to diabetes, cancer, and memory problems. Best of all, it's not a skimpy low-calorie regimen or no-fun, all-deprivation diet. Behind the program's satisfying meals is the latest nutrition and weight-loss research, harnessed to create an everyday eating plan in which virtually every food is a star, proven to help you lose weight and guard—or improve—your health. The guidelines:

A Wealth of Fruits, Vegetables, and Whole Grains
Serving guide: You'll eat two to four servings of fruit, four to six servings of vegetables, and four to six servings of grains every day—for a total of 50 to 60 percent of your daily calories.

The benefits: Low-glycemic carbohydrates—fresh fruits, vegetables, and whole grains—digest more slowly and release glucose to the bloodstream a little bit at a time over the course of hours. As a result, blood sugar and insulin (the hormone that tells cells to absorb blood sugar) stay lower. This reduces your health risks and, if your body is insulin-resistant (a common but often overlooked health problem in which your cells "ignore" signals from the insulin to absorb blood sugar), may also help you burn more fat when you're trying to lose weight.

Satisfying, Slimming Protein
Serving guide: You'll eat some protein at every meal, for a total of 15 to 25 percent of your daily calories.

The benefits: Getting enough protein as part of a weight-loss program may help shrink belly fat faster, Danish researchers say. The reason: Protein may inhibit the release of the stress hormone cortisol, which directs the body to store more fat in your abdomen. Losing belly fat is a great health move, because tummy fat is linked directly to prediabetic problems, diabetes itself, and heart disease. Protein can also help you lose weight by making you feel full and satisfied longer after a meal.

Low-Fat or Fat-Free Dairy

Serving guide: You'll eat two servings of dairy products on most days. (Dairy calories are counted as part of your daily quota of protein, fat, and even carbs, because milk contains all of these components.)

The benefits: Dairy foods not only help maintain bone density but may protect against metabolic syndrome, a prediabetic condition that raises your risk for heart attack, stroke, high blood pressure, type 2 diabetes, cancer, and memory loss. And if you haven't been getting enough calcium in your diet, adding dairy may help you lose weight more effectively, some research suggests. *Note:* Be sure to add a calcium supplement of about 500 milligrams per day to reach your recommended daily calcium intake of 1,000 to 1,200 milligrams.

Yummy "Good" Fats

Serving guide: You'll get 25 to 30 percent of your daily calories from fat—including daily servings of the good fats your body needs most.

The benefits: Early research suggests that getting plenty of omega-3s may cool chronic inflammation—a risk factor for metabolic syndrome and diabetes. Meanwhile, good fats have a proven track record as protectors against health problems brought on by metabolic syndrome. And the good fats in nuts (plus the fiber and protein) have helped dieters lose more weight in several studies.

Treats!

Serving guide: You'll enjoy one every day. On the menu: wine, desserts like chocolate chip cookies and brownies, snack foods such as whole grain tortilla chips, and low-fat ice cream.

The benefit: Desserts and appetizers featured in *Sugar Solution* recipes are cleverly designed to combine fats, fiber, and protein in a way that blunts the rise in blood sugar that usually accompanies dessert. Feeling pampered and satisfied isn't a luxury—it's a necessity that can help you stay on track. That's why a treat is included into every day of *Sugar Solution* eating. (Of course, practice moderation!)

STRATEGY #2: GET ACTIVE, GET FIT

Exercise gives you a burst of energy and helps you lose weight—plus, research shows that it's a powerful tool for keeping your blood sugar lower and steadier. Our three-step activity plan:

Walk! If you've never walked for fitness before, we'll show you how to start slowly for impressive results. By the end of the 28-day plan, walking rookies will be stepping out for 30 minutes of calorie-burning every day. Meanwhile, walking veterans will learn how to gradually ramp up to 60 minutes or more. (Feel free to substitute or mix and match other aerobic activities such as jogging, biking, swimming, cross-country skiing, or an exercise class or video.)

Strength-train! Nine simple exercises—most of which use only your body weight to work your muscles—tone you from head to toe. You can choose to do your strength training in 10-minute segments 6 days a week, 20-minute bouts 3 days a week, or 30 minutes just twice a week. It couldn't be more convenient—and you'll love the way this easy routine builds sleek muscle, whittles your waist, and slims your hips, while boosting your metabolism so you burn more calories all day, every day.

Incorporate everyday activity! In the past 50 years, modern technology has helped us engineer about 700 calories' worth of activity out of every single day. The *Sugar Solution* program will help you put more calorie-burning movement back into your day, wherever you can. Research shows that you can burn hundreds of extra calories every day this way, without ever changing into gym shorts and a T-shirt or scheduling exercise time on your calendar.

STRATEGY #3: SAY GOOD-BYE TO STRESS

We were so impressed by the growing body of research linking stress with weight gain, difficulty losing weight, and weight *regain*—as well as to high blood sugar and all of its related health problems—that we've made taming tension a key element of the *Sugar Solution* plan. De-stressing cannot take the place of a healthy diet or regular physical activity, but it *can* help you stick with the other elements of your program, achieve better results more swiftly, feel great right away, and insure that you've done all you can to sidestep blood sugar problems. If you already have above-normal blood sugar, stress reduction can also help bring your levels down. Our smart, stress-stopping strategies will help you:

• Develop resilience so that you rise above daily stresses

• Claim 15 minutes of "me time" a day for relaxation

• Pursue and enjoy pleasure in all its shapes and forms—every day

• Get plenty of deep, refreshing sleep

HOW TO USE THE *SUGAR SOLUTION* DAILY PLANNER

Two of the most powerful tools for making healthy lifestyle changes are a pen and a logbook. Experts say that when dieters write down their daily food choices, they're more likely to stay on track, feel more motivated to make healthy choices, and become aware more quickly of their personal danger zones. You also reap the rewards of seeing where your willpower and coping skills are strongest—and you might even notice areas where you're *under*eating! Same goes for exercise and stress reduction: Write it down, and you're more likely to follow through and admire your daily progress.

So grab a pen or pencil. Each week begins with a "Looking Ahead" page, where you'll find goals and inspiration for the next week, plus room to write down your own challenges and planned strategies. Each day of our 28-day program gets two pages—ample space for logging your food choices, exercise, lifestyle activities, and stress-soothing experiences. We've included special calorie-burning activities and spa-quality tranquility breaks, too. And at the end of each week, you'll find a "Review" page, where you can summarize your experience and log your current weight. (You can choose when to weigh in; just try to keep the day and time of your weigh-in consistent each week.) There's room to list your successes as well as your challenges, and don't hesitate to list both: Give yourself credit for every positive change, and don't be afraid to face your challenges. They're not faults—they're places where you're trying hard to grow and change!

My walking/aerobic exercise goal this week: Rookie, 15 minutes a day; veteran, 30 minutes a day or more

My strength-training goal this week: 10 minutes most days of the week

My active lifestyle goal this week: Get outside for fun or home/yard/car improvement projects at least once

My stress-reduction goal this week: A 5-minute soother in the morning, including 2 minutes of deep, slow breathing and 3 minutes thinking about everything you're grateful for

Sugar Solution Success Strategies for Week 1:

• Buy at least one "good fat" food at the grocery store this week, such as nuts, an avocado, or salmon. Enjoy!

• Remember to perform strength-training moves slo-o-owly. Count 2 to 4 seconds as you perform the first half of each exercise and another 2 to 4 as you do the second half. Your muscles will work harder, and you'll practice "perfect" form.

• Turn life into a mini workout. Walk to the mailbox to get the mail. March in place while chatting on the phone, or grab the cordless and walk around the house. Chores are an untapped source of calorie-burning activity!

Challenges I anticipate this week:

_____

_____

_____

Strategies I can use to overcome them:

_____

_____

_____

My goals for this week:

_____

_____

_____

_____

Check off each serving you eat of these *Sugar Solution* superfoods:

Fruit ☐ ☐ ☐ ☐

Vegetables ☐ ☐ ☐ ☐

Whole grains ☐ ☐ ☐ ☐ ☐ ☐ ☐

Low-fat or fat-free dairy products ☐ ☐ ☐

Good fats (in half-servings) ☑ ☑ ☑

Nuts (in half-servings) ☑

Lean protein (including eggs, lean meats, poultry, and tofu) ☐ ☐ ☐ ☐

Beans ☐ ☐

Water ☐ ☐ ☐ ☐ ☐ ☐ ☐

Tranquility Break

If you're laughing, it's hard to hold on to stress. Your facial muscles get a natural workout that relaxes them. Research shows that laughter can boost immunity, reduce pain, and protect your heart.

Splurges, extras, and oversize portions: _____
_____
_____

Best food choice today: _____
_____
_____

Exercise Log

Walking or other aerobic activity: _____ minutes

Strength training: Upper body ☐   Lower body ☐   Core ☐

My "lifestyle activity" choices included: _____
_____
_____

Stress-Soothing Check-In

My stress level today: Low ☐   Medium ☐   High ☐   Red Alert ☐

I reduced my stress by: _____
_____
_____

My thoughts and feelings about my food, exercise, and stress-relief choices today:

_____

_____

_____

_____

_____

_____

_____

_____

_____

_____

_____

_____

_____

_____

_____

_____

_____

_____

_____

_____

_____

_____

GET YOURSELF MOVING!

Grab your kids, your dog, and a Frisbee, and head to the park for half an hour.

Check off each serving you eat of these *Sugar Solution* superfoods:

Fruit ☐ ☐ ☐ ☐

Vegetables ☐ ☐ ☐ ☐

Whole grains ☐ ☐ ☐ ☐ ☐ ☐ ☐ ☐

Low-fat or fat-free dairy products ☐ ☐ ☐

Good fats (in half-servings) ☑ ☑ ☑

Nuts (in half-servings) ☑

Lean protein (including eggs, lean meats, poultry, and tofu) ☐ ☐ ☐ ☐

Beans ☐ ☐

Water ☐ ☐ ☐ ☐ ☐ ☐ ☐ ☐

Tranquility
Break

Take a bath before bed.
Soothing, warm water
(with a splash of
lavender bath oil)
cleanses away stress.

Splurges, extras, and oversize portions: _____

_____

_____

Best food choice today: _____

_____

_____

Exercise Log

Walking or other aerobic activity: _____ minutes

Strength training: Upper body ☐   Lower body ☐   Core ☐

My "lifestyle activity" choices included: _____

_____

_____

Stress-Soothing Check-In

My stress level today: Low ☐   Medium ☐   High ☐   Red Alert ☐

I reduced my stress by: _____

_____

_____

My thoughts and feelings about my food, exercise, and stress-relief choices today:

_____

_____

_____

_____

_____

_____

_____

_____

_____

_____

_____

_____

_____

_____

_____

_____

_____

_____

_____

_____

_____

GET YOURSELF MOVING!

Wash and wax your car yourself, by hand. You'll burn about 300 calories in an hour—and you'll have a nice shiny car to boot!

Check off each serving you eat of these *Sugar Solution* superfoods:

Fruit ☐ ☐ ☐ ☐

Vegetables ☐ ☐ ☐ ☐

Whole grains ☐ ☐ ☐ ☐ ☐ ☐ ☐

Low-fat or fat-free dairy products ☐ ☐ ☐

Good fats (in half-servings) ☑ ☑ ☑

Nuts (in half-servings) ☑

Lean protein (including eggs, lean meats, poultry, and tofu) ☐ ☐ ☐ ☐

Beans ☐ ☐

Water ☐ ☐ ☐ ☐ ☐ ☐ ☐

Tranquility Break

Breathe through your nose. Long, slow breathing soothes your parasympathetic nervous system and helps rest, restore, and expand the lower lungs.

Splurges, extras, and oversize portions: _____
_____
_____

Best food choice today: _____
_____
_____

Exercise Log

Walking or other aerobic activity: _____ minutes

Strength training: Upper body ☐   Lower body ☐   Core ☐

My "lifestyle activity" choices included: _____
_____
_____

Stress-Soothing Check-In

My stress level today: Low ☐   Medium ☐   High ☐   Red Alert ☐

I reduced my stress by: _____
_____
_____

My thoughts and feelings about my food, exercise, and stress-relief choices today:

_____

_____

_____

_____

_____

_____

_____

_____

_____

_____

_____

_____

_____

_____

_____

_____

_____

_____

_____

_____

_____

_____

GET YOURSELF MOVING!

If it's a nice day outside, hang your laundry on your clothesline (if you can still find your old clothespins). Remember how good line-dried T-shirts smell?

Check off each serving you eat of these *Sugar Solution* superfoods:

Fruit ☐ ☐ ☐ ☐

Vegetables ☐ ☐ ☐ ☐

Whole grains ☐ ☐ ☐ ☐ ☐ ☐ ☐

Low-fat or fat-free dairy products ☐ ☐ ☐

Good fats (in half-servings) ☑ ☑ ☑

Nuts (in half-servings) ☑

Lean protein (including eggs, lean meats, poultry, and tofu) ☐ ☐ ☐ ☐

Beans ☐ ☐

Water ☐ ☐ ☐ ☐ ☐ ☐ ☐ ☐

Tranquility Break

Remember to say no. When life gets tough, don't take on extra chores and responsibilities that aren't 100 percent essential.

Splurges, extras, and oversize portions: _____
_____
_____

Best food choice today: _____
_____
_____

Exercise Log

Walking or other aerobic activity: _____ minutes

Strength training: Upper body ☐   Lower body ☐   Core ☐

My "lifestyle activity" choices included: _____
_____
_____

Stress-Soothing Check-In

My stress level today: Low ☐   Medium ☐   High ☐   Red Alert ☐

I reduced my stress by: _____
_____
_____

My thoughts and feelings about my food, exercise, and stress-relief choices today:

_____

_____

_____

_____

_____

_____

_____

_____

_____

_____

_____

_____

_____

_____

_____

_____

_____

_____

_____

_____

_____

_____

_____

GET YOURSELF MOVING!

Close the shades, crank up the tunes, and dance like crazy—after all, there's no one watching.

Check off each serving you eat of these *Sugar Solution* superfoods:

Fruit ☐ ☐ ☐ ☐

Vegetables ☐ ☐ ☐ ☐

Whole grains ☐ ☐ ☐ ☐ ☐ ☐ ☐ ☐

Low-fat or fat-free dairy products ☐ ☐ ☐

Good fats (in half-servings) ☑ ☑ ☑

Nuts (in half-servings) ☑

Lean protein (including eggs, lean meats, poultry, and tofu) ☐ ☐ ☐ ☐

Beans ☐ ☐

Water ☐ ☐ ☐ ☐ ☐ ☐ ☐ ☐

Tranquility Break

Get perspective. Feeling crazy? Ask yourself, Is this a life-and-death matter or everyday stress? It will pass.

Splurges, extras, and oversize portions: _____
_____
_____

Best food choice today: _____
_____
_____

Exercise Log

Walking or other aerobic activity: _____ minutes

Strength training: Upper body ☐   Lower body ☐   Core ☐

My "lifestyle activity" choices included: _____
_____
_____

Stress-Soothing Check-In

My stress level today: Low ☐   Medium ☐   High ☐   Red Alert ☐

I reduced my stress by: _____
_____
_____

My thoughts and feelings about my food, exercise, and stress-relief choices today:

_____

_____

_____

_____

_____

_____

_____

_____

_____

_____

_____

_____

_____

_____

_____

_____

_____

_____

_____

_____

_____

_____

_____

GET YOURSELF MOVING!

Do 30 minutes of weeding or other yard work, either at your own home or an elderly neighbor's.

Check off each serving you eat of these *Sugar Solution* superfoods:

Fruit ☐ ☐ ☐ ☐

Vegetables ☐ ☐ ☐ ☐

Whole grains ☐ ☐ ☐ ☐ ☐ ☐ ☐ ☐

Low-fat or fat-free dairy products ☐ ☐ ☐

Good fats (in half-servings) ☑ ☑ ☑

Nuts (in half-servings) ☑

Lean protein (including eggs, lean meats, poultry, and tofu) ☐ ☐ ☐ ☐

Beans ☐ ☐

Water ☐ ☐ ☐ ☐ ☐ ☐ ☐ ☐

Tranquility Break

Think before you blurt. Feeling angry with your spouse, the kids, a co-worker or neighbor? Analyze your emotions before you speak. Pay attention to how you're body's feeling, get comfortable, then consider a calm response.

Splurges, extras, and oversize portions: _____

_____

_____

Best food choice today: _____

_____

_____

Exercise Log

Walking or other aerobic activity: _____ minutes

Strength training: Upper body ☐   Lower body ☐   Core ☐

My "lifestyle activity" choices included: _____

_____

_____

Stress-Soothing Check-In

My stress level today: Low ☐   Medium ☐   High ☐   Red Alert ☐

I reduced my stress by: _____

_____

_____

My thoughts and feelings about my food, exercise, and stress-relief choices today:

_____

_____

_____

_____

_____

_____

_____

_____

_____

_____

_____

_____

_____

_____

_____

_____

_____

_____

_____

GET YOURSELF MOVING!

Going to the mall? Do one brisk lap around the perimeter before you start shopping. See if you can do another lap after your errands are done.

Check off each serving you eat of these *Sugar Solution* superfoods:

Fruit ☐ ☐ ☐ ☐

Vegetables ☐ ☐ ☐ ☐

Whole grains ☐ ☐ ☐ ☐ ☐ ☐ ☐

Low-fat or fat-free dairy products ☐ ☐ ☐

Good fats (in half-servings) ☑ ☑ ☑

Nuts (in half-servings) ☑

Lean protein (including eggs, lean meats, poultry, and tofu) ☐ ☐ ☐ ☐

Beans ☐ ☐

Water ☐ ☐ ☐ ☐ ☐ ☐ ☐ ☐

Tranquility Break

You can win 90 percent of the time; 10 percent of the time, you can't. That's the time to surrender. It's somebody else's turn to win.

Splurges, extras, and oversize portions: _____

_____

_____

Best food choice today: _____

_____

_____

Exercise Log

Walking or other aerobic activity: _____ minutes

Strength training: Upper body ☐   Lower body ☐   Core ☐

My "lifestyle activity" choices included: _____

_____

_____

Stress-Soothing Check-In

My stress level today: Low ☐   Medium ☐   High ☐   Red Alert ☐

I reduced my stress by: _____

_____

_____

My thoughts and feelings about my food, exercise, and stress-relief choices today:

_____

_____

_____

_____

_____

_____

_____

_____

_____

_____

_____

_____

_____

_____

_____

_____

_____

_____

_____

_____

GET YOURSELF MOVING!

Do as many errands as you can on foot today. For example, instead of driving to your neighborhood pharmacy after work, patronize the drugstore that's within walking distance of your office. If you live in an area with shops close by, walk a few extra blocks to try someplace new.

WEEK 1 REVIEW

DATE _____ DAY _____

My weight at the end of the week: _____ Weight change this week: _____

Biggest successes and choices I'm most proud of regarding . . .

Diet: _____

_____

Exercise: _____

_____

Stress reduction: _____

_____

Biggest challenges this week—and how I met them—regarding . . .

Diet: _____

_____

Exercise: _____

_____

Stress reduction: _____

_____

Lessons I learned this week:

_____

_____

_____

_____

Patterns I noticed this week related to eating, exercise, or stress:

_____

_____

_____

_____

_____

My walking/aerobic exercise goal this week: Rookie, 20 minutes a day; veteran, 40 minutes a day or more

My strength-training goal this week: Continue with 10 minutes most days of the week. Try combining two of the three routines, then taking the next day off.

My active lifestyle goal this week: Get outside twice this week for active fun or some calorie-burning outdoor chores.

My stress-reduction goal this week: Continue with your 5-minute morning soother; add a brief meditation (follow your breath as you sit comfortably, eyes closed, for 5 minutes) in the evening.

Sugar Solution Success Strategies for Week 2:

• Got kids or grandkids? Stock a box with a kickball, chalk for making hopscotch squares, a Frisbee, a wiffle ball and bat, a hula hoop, and a croquet or bocce set. Now get out there!

• Check your shoes. Replace walking shoes about every 10 months. Wear athletic socks to the store, and take a test walk before you buy. The best choice will leave room at the toe for your foot to expand and will be flat—your heel and the ball of your foot should be at about the same level.

• Buy a pretty water bottle—and carry it every day. Aim to sip eight 8-ounce cups' worth every 24 hours.

Challenges I anticipate this week:

_____

_____

_____

Strategies I can use to overcome them:

_____

_____

_____

My goals for this week:

_____

_____

_____

Check off each serving you eat of these *Sugar Solution* superfoods:

Fruit ☐ ☐ ☐ ☐

Vegetables ☐ ☐ ☐ ☐

Whole grains ☐ ☐ ☐ ☐ ☐ ☐ ☐

Low-fat or fat-free dairy products ☐ ☐ ☐

Good fats (in half-servings) ☑ ☑ ☑

Nuts (in half-servings) ☑

Lean protein (including eggs, lean meats, poultry, and tofu) ☐ ☐ ☐ ☐

Beans ☐ ☐

Water ☐ ☐ ☐ ☐ ☐ ☐ ☐ ☐

Tranquility Break

Practice optimism. Fight the urge to give in to hopelessness, helplessness, and defeat. Regroup, stay positive, and look for solutions.

Splurges, extras, and oversize portions: _____

_____

_____

Best food choice today: _____

_____

_____

Exercise Log

Walking or other aerobic activity: _____ minutes

Strength training: Upper body ☐   Lower body ☐   Core ☐

My "lifestyle activity" choices included: _____

_____

_____

Stress-Soothing Check-In

My stress level today: Low ☐   Medium ☐   High ☐   Red Alert ☐

I reduced my stress by: _____

_____

_____

My thoughts and feelings about my food, exercise, and stress-relief choices today:

_____

_____

_____

_____

_____

_____

_____

_____

_____

_____

_____

_____

_____

_____

_____

_____

_____

_____

_____

_____

GET YOURSELF MOVING!

Go bowling and stand while you wait your turn on the lane. Eat a healthful meal or snack before you head to the alley so you won't be tempted by the snack bar.

Check off each serving you eat of these *Sugar Solution* superfoods:

Fruit	☐ ☐ ☐ ☐
Vegetables	☐ ☐ ☐ ☐
Whole grains	☐ ☐ ☐ ☐ ☐ ☐ ☐
Low-fat or fat-free dairy products	☐ ☐ ☐
Good fats (in half-servings)	☑ ☑ ☑
Nuts (in half-servings)	☑
Lean protein (including eggs, lean meats, poultry, and tofu)	☐ ☐ ☐ ☐
Beans	☐ ☐
Water	☐ ☐ ☐ ☐ ☐ ☐ ☐

Tranquility Break

High-stress situation? Don't give in to distraction. When you're stressed-out, you can let your guard down. Pamper yourself, take your time, have a cup of tea—and stay focused.

Splurges, extras, and oversize portions: _____
_____
_____

Best food choice today: _____
_____
_____

Exercise Log

Walking or other aerobic activity: _____ minutes

Strength training: Upper body ☐   Lower body ☐   Core ☐

My "lifestyle activity" choices included: _____
_____
_____

Stress-Soothing Check-In

My stress level today: Low ☐   Medium ☐   High ☐   Red Alert ☐

I reduced my stress by: _____
_____
_____

My thoughts and feelings about my food, exercise, and stress-relief choices today:

_____

_____

_____

_____

_____

_____

_____

_____

_____

_____

_____

_____

_____

_____

_____

_____

_____

_____

_____

_____

GET YOURSELF MOVING!

Pick up a jump rope and use it. You'll feel 8 years old again. Jump just high enough to clear the rope, and bend your knees slightly when you land. This will minimize the impact on your knees.

Check off each serving you eat of these *Sugar Solution* superfoods:

Fruit ☐ ☐ ☐ ☐

Vegetables ☐ ☐ ☐ ☐

Whole grains ☐ ☐ ☐ ☐ ☐ ☐ ☐ ☐

Low-fat or fat-free dairy products ☐ ☐ ☐

Good fats (in half-servings) ☑ ☑ ☑

Nuts (in half-servings) ☑

Lean protein (including eggs, lean meats, poultry, and tofu) ☐ ☐ ☐ ☐

Beans ☐ ☐

Water ☐ ☐ ☐ ☐ ☐ ☐ ☐ ☐

Tranquility Break

Give it your all, then let go. Things not going right? Do your best, remind yourself that you've done your best, then step back. No second thoughts necessary.

Splurges, extras, and oversize portions: _____
_____
_____

Best food choice today: _____
_____
_____

Exercise Log

Walking or other aerobic activity: _____ minutes

Strength training: Upper body ☐   Lower body ☐   Core ☐

My "lifestyle activity" choices included: _____
_____
_____

Stress-Soothing Check-In

My stress level today: Low ☐   Medium ☐   High ☐   Red Alert ☐

I reduced my stress by: _____
_____
_____

My thoughts and feelings about my food, exercise, and stress-relief choices today:

_____

_____

_____

_____

_____

_____

_____

_____

_____

_____

_____

_____

_____

_____

_____

_____

_____

_____

_____

_____

_____

_____

GET YOURSELF MOVING!

If you normally let the bagger load your groceries into your car, do it yourself today. Leave your cart near the entrance and make several trips, if necessary.

Check off each serving you eat of these *Sugar Solution* superfoods:

Fruit ☐ ☐ ☐ ☐

Vegetables ☐ ☐ ☐ ☐

Whole grains ☐ ☐ ☐ ☐ ☐ ☐ ☐

Low-fat or fat-free dairy products ☐ ☐ ☐

Good fats (in half-servings) ☑ ☑ ☑

Nuts (in half-servings) ☑

Lean protein (including eggs, lean meats, poultry, and tofu) ☐ ☐ ☐ ☐

Beans ☐ ☐

Water ☐ ☐ ☐ ☐ ☐ ☐ ☐

Tranquility Break

Honor your own needs. Caregiving? Working long hours? Lots of extra responsibilities right now? Don't give up your de-stressing time— whether it's exercise, 15 minutes of yoga, or tug- of-war with your dog.

Splurges, extras, and oversize portions: _____

_____

_____

Best food choice today: _____

_____

_____

Exercise Log

Walking or other aerobic activity: _____ minutes

Strength training: Upper body ☐   Lower body ☐   Core ☐

My "lifestyle activity" choices included: _____

_____

_____

Stress-Soothing Check-In

My stress level today: Low ☐   Medium ☐   High ☐   Red Alert ☐

I reduced my stress by: _____

_____

_____

My thoughts and feelings about my food, exercise, and stress-relief choices today:

_____

_____

_____

_____

_____

_____

_____

_____

_____

_____

_____

_____

_____

_____

_____

_____

_____

_____

_____

_____

_____

_____

_____

GET YOURSELF MOVING!

Stand up straight. You'll burn more calories and look taller and slimmer to boot.

Check off each serving you eat of these *Sugar Solution* superfoods:

Fruit ☐ ☐ ☐ ☐

Vegetables ☐ ☐ ☐ ☐

Whole grains ☐ ☐ ☐ ☐ ☐ ☐ ☐

Low-fat or fat-free dairy products ☐ ☐ ☐

Good fats (in half-servings) ☑ ☑ ☑

Nuts (in half-servings) ☑

Lean protein (including eggs, lean meats, poultry, and tofu) ☐ ☐ ☐ ☐

Beans ☐ ☐

Water ☐ ☐ ☐ ☐ ☐ ☐ ☐ ☐

> *Tranquility Break*
>
> *Get into the kitchen. The creative act of preparing wonderful food—chopping vegetables, cooking, adding pungent seasonings, and, finally, eating a great meal—is food for the soul.*

Splurges, extras, and oversize portions: _____
_____
_____

Best food choice today: _____
_____
_____

Exercise Log

Walking or other aerobic activity: _____ minutes

Strength training: Upper body ☐   Lower body ☐   Core ☐

My "lifestyle activity" choices included: _____
_____
_____

Stress-Soothing Check-In

My stress level today: Low ☐   Medium ☐   High ☐   Red Alert ☐

I reduced my stress by: _____
_____
_____

My thoughts and feelings about my food, exercise, and stress-relief choices today:

_____

_____

_____

_____

_____

_____

_____

_____

_____

_____

_____

_____

_____

_____

_____

_____

_____

_____

_____

_____

_____

_____

GET YOURSELF MOVING!

Borrow, rent, or buy an exercise video that you've never tried before—and use it.

Check off each serving you eat of these *Sugar Solution* superfoods:

Fruit □ □ □ □

Vegetables □ □ □ □

Whole grains □ □ □ □ □ □ □ □

Low-fat or fat-free dairy products □ □ □

Good fats (in half-servings) ☑ ☑ ☑

Nuts (in half-servings) ☑

Lean protein (including eggs, lean meats, poultry, and tofu) □ □ □ □

Beans □ □

Water □ □ □ □ □ □ □ □

Tranquility Break

Soothe yourself through music. The number one thing most people around the world do when they're stressed-out is listen to music, reports a poll by Roper Starch Worldwide.

Splurges, extras, and oversize portions: _____
_____
_____

Best food choice today: _____
_____
_____

Exercise Log

Walking or other aerobic activity: _____ minutes

Strength training: Upper body □   Lower body □   Core □

My "lifestyle activity" choices included: _____
_____
_____

Stress-Soothing Check-In

My stress level today: Low □   Medium □   High □   Red Alert □

I reduced my stress by: _____
_____
_____

My thoughts and feelings about my food, exercise, and stress-relief choices today:

_____

_____

_____

_____

_____

_____

_____

_____

_____

_____

_____

_____

_____

_____

_____

_____

_____

_____

_____

_____

_____

_____

_____

_____

GET YOURSELF MOVING!

Go ice skating or in-line skating. If you don't know how, go anyway (equipped with a helmet and knee and elbow pads, if you're inline skating), and burn calories trying to stay upright.

Check off each serving you eat of these *Sugar Solution* superfoods:

Fruit ☐ ☐ ☐ ☐

Vegetables ☐ ☐ ☐ ☐

Whole grains ☐ ☐ ☐ ☐ ☐ ☐ ☐

Low-fat or fat-free dairy products ☐ ☐ ☐

Good fats (in half-servings) ☑ ☑ ☑

Nuts (in half-servings) ☑

Lean protein (including eggs, lean meats, poultry, and tofu) ☐ ☐ ☐ ☐

Beans ☐ ☐

Water ☐ ☐ ☐ ☐ ☐ ☐ ☐ ☐

Tranquility Break

Breathe through your belly. Blow all the breath out of your lungs, then focus on a point about 2 inches below your navel, in the center of your body. Inhale, feeling your entire belly expand. Then breathe out slowly. Do this 10 times.

Splurges, extras, and oversize portions: _____

_____

_____

Best food choice today: _____

_____

_____

Exercise Log

Walking or other aerobic activity: _____ minutes

Strength training: Upper body ☐   Lower body ☐   Core ☐

My "lifestyle activity" choices included: _____

_____

_____

Stress-Soothing Check-In

My stress level today: Low ☐   Medium ☐   High ☐   Red Alert ☐

I reduced my stress by: _____

_____

_____

My thoughts and feelings about my food, exercise, and stress-relief choices today:

_____

_____

_____

_____

_____

_____

_____

_____

_____

_____

_____

_____

_____

_____

_____

_____

_____

_____

_____

_____

_____

_____

_____

GET YOURSELF MOVING!

Suggest a walking meeting at work. Physical activity can help generate creative ideas, and meetings will be more stimulating and productive.

WEEK 2 REVIEW

DATE _____ DAY _____

My weight at the end of the week: _____ Weight change this week: _____

Biggest successes and choices I'm most proud of regarding . . .

Diet: _____

_____

Exercise: _____

_____

Stress reduction: _____

_____

Biggest challenges this week—and how I met them—regarding . . .

Diet: _____

_____

Exercise: _____

_____

Stress reduction: _____

_____

Lessons I learned this week:

_____

_____

_____

_____

Patterns I noticed this week related to eating, exercise, or stress:

_____

_____

_____

_____

_____

My walking/aerobic exercise goal this week: Rookie, 25 minutes a day; veteran, 50 minutes a day or more

My strength-training goal this week: 10 minutes most days. Look over your schedule for the week, and plan ahead for busy days: Do a longer routine a day ahead so you can take off on busy days without losing exercise time.

My active lifestyle goal this week: Get extra activity at least twice this week.

My stress-reduction goal this week: Turn off the TV and hang up the phone. Go to bed a half hour earlier.

Sugar Solution **Success Strategies for Week 3:**

• Don't underestimate the calorie-burning potential of chores. A half hour of TV watching burns a piddling 37 calories. In contrast, 30 minutes spent in these chores will burn nearly 200 calories: painting the house, washing the car, gardening, raking leaves, shoveling snow.

• Explore the produce department. Find one new fruit to take home and try. We love mangoes, pomegranates, and star fruit.

• Buy, cut, or pick a pretty bouquet. Several studies show that looking at colorful blooms eases stress.

Challenges I anticipate this week:

_____

_____

_____

Strategies I can use to overcome them:

_____

_____

_____

My goals for this week:

_____

_____

_____

DATE _____ **DAY** _____

Check off each serving you eat of these *Sugar Solution* superfoods:

Fruit ☐ ☐ ☐ ☐

Vegetables ☐ ☐ ☐ ☐

Whole grains ☐ ☐ ☐ ☐ ☐ ☐ ☐

Low-fat or fat-free dairy products ☐ ☐ ☐

Good fats (in half-servings) ☑ ☑ ☑

Nuts (in half-servings) ☑

Lean protein (including eggs, lean meats, poultry, and tofu) ☐ ☐ ☐ ☐

Beans ☐ ☐

Water ☐ ☐ ☐ ☐ ☐ ☐ ☐

Tranquility Break

Give up the shoulder hunch. Tense muscles ramp up anxiety and negative thinking. Escape by relaxing your muscles consciously each time you exhale.

Splurges, extras, and oversize portions: _____

_____

Best food choice today: _____

_____

Exercise Log

Walking or other aerobic activity: _____ minutes

Strength training: Upper body ☐   Lower body ☐   Core ☐

My "lifestyle activity" choices included: _____

_____

Stress-Soothing Check-In

My stress level today: Low ☐   Medium ☐   High ☐   Red Alert ☐

I reduced my stress by: _____

_____

My thoughts and feelings about my food, exercise, and stress-relief choices today:

_____

_____

_____

_____

_____

_____

_____

_____

_____

_____

_____

_____

_____

_____

_____

_____

_____

_____

_____

_____

GET YOURSELF MOVING!

Make a list of 15-minute walks you can do from home or work. When you find yourself with a sliver of time, head out for a quick perk-me-up.

Check off each serving you eat of these *Sugar Solution* superfoods:

Fruit   ☐ ☐ ☐ ☐

Vegetables   ☐ ☐ ☐ ☐

Whole grains   ☐ ☐ ☐ ☐ ☐ ☐ ☐

Low-fat or fat-free dairy products   ☐ ☐ ☐

Good fats (in half-servings)   ☑ ☑ ☑

Nuts (in half-servings)   ☑

Lean protein (including eggs, lean meats, poultry, and tofu)   ☐ ☐ ☐ ☐

Beans   ☐ ☐

Water   ☐ ☐ ☐ ☐ ☐ ☐ ☐

Tranquility Break

Put on a happy face. Forty percent of us have "smile muscles"—using them sends a happy message to your brain. Are you one of them? Try it!

Splurges, extras, and oversize portions: _____

_____

_____

Best food choice today: _____

_____

_____

Exercise Log

Walking or other aerobic activity: _____ minutes

Strength training: Upper body ☐   Lower body ☐   Core ☐

My "lifestyle activity" choices included: _____

_____

_____

Stress-Soothing Check-In

My stress level today: Low ☐   Medium ☐   High ☐   Red Alert ☐

I reduced my stress by: _____

_____

_____

My thoughts and feelings about my food, exercise, and stress-relief choices today:

_____

_____

_____

_____

_____

_____

_____

_____

_____

_____

_____

_____

_____

_____

_____

_____

_____

_____

_____

_____

GET YOURSELF MOVING!

Instead of taking the elevator two or three floors, take the stairs. Or, if you ride upstairs, walk back down.

Check off each serving you eat of these *Sugar Solution* superfoods:

Fruit ☐ ☐ ☐ ☐

Vegetables ☐ ☐ ☐ ☐

Whole grains ☐ ☐ ☐ ☐ ☐ ☐ ☐ ☐

Low-fat or fat-free dairy products ☐ ☐ ☐

Good fats (in half-servings) ☑ ☑ ☑

Nuts (in half-servings) ☑

Lean protein (including eggs, lean meats, poultry, and tofu) ☐ ☐ ☐ ☐

Beans ☐ ☐

Water ☐ ☐ ☐ ☐ ☐ ☐ ☐ ☐

Tranquility Break

Keep a bottle of a pleasing aromatherapy scent handy: peppermint for a pick-me-up; lavender and rose for relaxation. A spritz activates olfactory structures in the brain where emotions are processed.

Splurges, extras, and oversize portions: _____

_____

_____

Best food choice today: _____

_____

_____

Exercise Log

Walking or other aerobic activity: _____ minutes

Strength training: Upper body ☐   Lower body ☐   Core ☐

My "lifestyle activity" choices included: _____

_____

_____

Stress-Soothing Check-In

My stress level today: Low ☐   Medium ☐   High ☐   Red Alert ☐

I reduced my stress by: _____

_____

_____

My thoughts and feelings about my food, exercise, and stress-relief choices today:

_____

_____

_____

_____

_____

_____

_____

_____

_____

_____

_____

_____

_____

_____

_____

_____

_____

_____

_____

_____

_____

_____

GET YOURSELF MOVING!

Instead of using the garage-door opener, get out of your car and open the door yourself.

Check off each serving you eat of these *Sugar Solution* superfoods:

Fruit					☐	☐	☐	☐
Vegetables					☐	☐	☐	☐
Whole grains		☐	☐	☐	☐	☐	☐	☐
Low-fat or fat-free dairy products						☐	☐	☐
Good fats (in half-servings)						☑	☑	☑
Nuts (in half-servings)								☑
Lean protein (including eggs, lean meats, poultry, and tofu)					☐	☐	☐	☐
Beans							☐	☐
Water		☐	☐	☐	☐	☐	☐	☐

Tranquility Break

Try yoga. This healing Eastern exercise diminished stress symptoms in a 2004 study of 18 yoga students.

Splurges, extras, and oversize portions: _____
_____
_____

Best food choice today: _____
_____
_____

Exercise Log

Walking or other aerobic activity: _____ minutes

Strength training: Upper body ☐   Lower body ☐   Core ☐

My "lifestyle activity" choices included: _____
_____
_____

Stress-Soothing Check-In

My stress level today: Low ☐   Medium ☐   High ☐   Red Alert ☐

I reduced my stress by: _____
_____
_____

My thoughts and feelings about my food, exercise, and stress-relief choices today:

_____

_____

_____

_____

_____

_____

_____

_____

_____

_____

_____

_____

_____

_____

_____

_____

_____

_____

_____

_____

_____

_____

GET YOURSELF MOVING!

Instead of sending e-mail to your colleagues, get up and walk to their offices. (You may want to call ahead to make sure you don't interrupt them.)

Check off each serving you eat of these *Sugar Solution* superfoods:

Fruit ☐ ☐ ☐ ☐

Vegetables ☐ ☐ ☐ ☐

Whole grains ☐ ☐ ☐ ☐ ☐ ☐ ☐

Low-fat or fat-free dairy products ☐ ☐ ☐

Good fats (in half-servings) ☒ ☒ ☒

Nuts (in half-servings) ☒

Lean protein (including eggs, lean meats, poultry, and tofu) ☐ ☐ ☐ ☐

Beans ☐ ☐

Water ☐ ☐ ☐ ☐ ☐ ☐ ☐

> ## *Tranquility Break*
>
> *Let your computer say om. Find—or create—a screen saver with a beautiful scene that relaxes you, or use words that help you feel centered and joyful. We like* faith, family, love, *and* joy.

Splurges, extras, and oversize portions: _____

_____

_____

Best food choice today: _____

_____

_____

Exercise Log

Walking or other aerobic activity: _____ minutes

Strength training: Upper body ☐   Lower body ☐   Core ☐

My "lifestyle activity" choices included: _____

_____

_____

Stress-Soothing Check-In

My stress level today: Low ☐   Medium ☐   High ☐   Red Alert ☐

I reduced my stress by: _____

_____

_____

My thoughts and feelings about my food, exercise, and stress-relief choices today:

_____

_____

_____

_____

_____

_____

_____

_____

_____

_____

_____

_____

_____

_____

_____

_____

_____

_____

_____

_____

_____

_____

_____

_____

GET YOURSELF MOVING!

When nature calls, don't use the nearest facilities. At home or at work, use the bathroom that's a floor above or below you.

Check off each serving you eat of these *Sugar Solution* superfoods:

Fruit ☐ ☐ ☐ ☐

Vegetables ☐ ☐ ☐ ☐

Whole grains ☐ ☐ ☐ ☐ ☐ ☐ ☐

Low-fat or fat-free dairy products ☐ ☐ ☐

Good fats (in half-servings) ☑ ☑ ☑

Nuts (in half-servings) ☑

Lean protein (including eggs, lean meats, poultry, and tofu) ☐ ☐ ☐ ☐

Beans ☐ ☐

Water ☐ ☐ ☐ ☐ ☐ ☐ ☐

Tranquility Break

Invent a new soother. Skip the Twinkies. When you're stressed, give yourself (or schedule) a manicure, pedicure, or even a shampoo with a gloriously scented new shampoo. Ahhh.

Splurges, extras, and oversize portions: _____

_____

_____

Best food choice today: _____

_____

_____

Exercise Log

Walking or other aerobic activity: _____ minutes

Strength training: Upper body ☐   Lower body ☐   Core ☐

My "lifestyle activity" choices included: _____

_____

_____

Stress-Soothing Check-In

My stress level today: Low ☐   Medium ☐   High ☐   Red Alert ☐

I reduced my stress by: _____

_____

_____

My thoughts and feelings about my food, exercise, and stress-relief choices today:

_____

_____

_____

_____

_____

_____

_____

_____

_____

_____

_____

_____

_____

_____

_____

_____

_____

_____

_____

_____

_____

_____

GET YOURSELF MOVING!

Instead of paying at the pump, get out of your car and walk in to pay the attendant at the station.

Check off each serving you eat of these *Sugar Solution* superfoods:

Fruit ☐ ☐ ☐ ☐

Vegetables ☐ ☐ ☐ ☐ ☐

Whole grains ☐ ☐ ☐ ☐ ☐ ☐ ☐ ☐

Low-fat or fat-free dairy products ☐ ☐ ☐

Good fats (in half-servings) ☑ ☑ ☑

Nuts (in half-servings) ☑

Lean protein (including eggs, lean meats, poultry, and tofu) ☐ ☐ ☐ ☐

Beans ☐ ☐

Water ☐ ☐ ☐ ☐ ☐ ☐ ☐ ☐

Tranquility Break

Make time for friends. Research shows that women's number one response to stress is to get together with other women. Invite a friend on your daily walk, make time for coffee and conversation, or call an old buddy on the phone.

Splurges, extras, and oversize portions: _____

_____

_____

Best food choice today: _____

_____

_____

Exercise Log

Walking or other aerobic activity: _____ minutes

Strength training: Upper body ☐   Lower body ☐   Core ☐

My "lifestyle activity" choices included: _____

_____

_____

Stress-Soothing Check-In

My stress level today: Low ☐   Medium ☐   High ☐   Red Alert ☐

I reduced my stress by: _____

_____

_____

My thoughts and feelings about my food, exercise, and stress-relief choices today:

_____

_____

_____

_____

_____

_____

_____

_____

_____

_____

_____

_____

_____

_____

_____

_____

_____

_____

_____

_____

_____

GET YOURSELF MOVING!

Instead of shopping online, shop at the mall. Of course, park your car far away from your preferred entrance.

WEEK 3 REVIEW

DATE _____ DAY_____

My weight at the end of the week: _____ Weight change this week: _____

My biggest successes and choices I'm most proud of regarding . . .

Diet: _____

_____

Exercise: _____

_____

Stress reduction: _____

_____

Biggest challenges this week—and how I met them—regarding . . .

Diet: _____

_____

Exercise: _____

_____

Stress reduction: _____

_____

Lessons I learned this week:

_____

_____

_____

_____

Patterns I noticed this week related to eating, exercise, or stress:

_____

_____

_____

_____

_____

My walking/aerobic exercise goal this week: Rookie, 30 minutes a day; veteran, 50 minutes a day

My strength-training goal this week: Keep it up! Consider switching to slightly heavier weights if you can effortlessly lift what you're now using. For moves without weights, add more repetitions if the exercises seem too easy.

My active lifestyle goal this week: Three activities. These can include a major housecleaning or yard-work project, energetic fun with the kids, roller-skating or bowling, or even a serious walk around the mall before shopping.

My stress-reduction goal this week: Enjoy an inspiring, soothing walk. On one of your daily treks, focus on taking calm breaths. Choose a beautiful park, neighborhood, or road. Admire the scenery around you.

Challenges I anticipate this week:

_____

_____

_____

Strategies I can use to overcome them:

_____

_____

_____

My goals for this week:

_____

_____

_____

Check off each serving you eat of these *Sugar Solution* superfoods:

Fruit □ □ □ □

Vegetables □ □ □ □

Whole grains □ □ □ □ □ □ □

Low-fat or fat-free dairy products □ □ □

Good fats (in half-servings) ☑ ☑ ☑

Nuts (in half-servings) ☑

Lean protein (including eggs, lean meats, poultry, and tofu) □ □ □ □

Beans □ □

Water □ □ □ □ □ □ □

Tranquility Break

Write yourself a letter. Feeling mad? Bad? Compose a quick note to yourself—or to the object of your dark feelings—but don't send it. The point is to figure out what's really upsetting you.

Splurges, extras, and oversize portions: _____

_____

_____

Best food choice today: _____

_____

_____

Exercise Log

Walking or other aerobic activity: _____ minutes

Strength training: Upper body □   Lower body □   Core □

My "lifestyle activity" choices included: _____

_____

_____

Stress-Soothing Check-In

My stress level today: Low □   Medium □   High □   Red Alert □

I reduced my stress by: _____

_____

_____

My thoughts and feelings about my food, exercise, and stress-relief choices today:

_____

_____

_____

_____

_____

_____

_____

_____

_____

_____

_____

_____

_____

_____

_____

_____

_____

_____

_____

_____

_____

GET YOURSELF MOVING!

For today's workout, head for the hills. Whether you're walking, running, or biking, propelling yourself uphill adds extra oomph to a cardio workout.

Check off each serving you eat of these *Sugar Solution* superfoods:

Fruit ☐ ☐ ☐ ☐

Vegetables ☐ ☐ ☐ ☐

Whole grains ☐ ☐ ☐ ☐ ☐ ☐ ☐

Low-fat or fat-free dairy products ☐ ☐ ☐

Good fats (in half-servings) ☑ ☑ ☑

Nuts (in half-servings) ☑

Lean protein (including eggs, lean meats, poultry, and tofu) ☐ ☐ ☐ ☐

Beans ☐ ☐

Water ☐ ☐ ☐ ☐ ☐ ☐ ☐

Tranquility Break

Revive old-fashioned downtime: Read the newspaper. Do a crossword puzzle. Sew on a button. Sit on the patio with a glass of iced tea and listen to the birds sing. Play Scrabble with your spouse or a friend.

Splurges, extras, and oversize portions: _____

_____

_____

Best food choice today: _____

_____

_____

Exercise Log

Walking or other aerobic activity: _____ minutes

Strength training: Upper body ☐   Lower body ☐   Core ☐

My "lifestyle activity" choices included: _____

_____

_____

Stress-Soothing Check-In

My stress level today: Low ☐   Medium ☐   High ☐   Red Alert ☐

I reduced my stress by: _____

_____

_____

My thoughts and feelings about my food, exercise, and stress-relief choices today:

_____

_____

_____

_____

_____

_____

_____

_____

_____

_____

_____

_____

_____

_____

_____

_____

_____

_____

_____

_____

_____

_____

GET YOURSELF MOVING!

Instead of reclining on the couch or in your office chair while you talk on the phone, get up and walk around your living room or office.

Check off each serving you eat of these *Sugar Solution* superfoods:

Fruit ☐ ☐ ☐ ☐

Vegetables ☐ ☐ ☐ ☐ ☐

Whole grains ☐ ☐ ☐ ☐ ☐ ☐ ☐ ☐

Low-fat or fat-free dairy products ☐ ☐ ☐

Good fats (in half-servings) ☒ ☒ ☒

Nuts (in half-servings) ☒

Lean protein (including eggs, lean meats, poultry, and tofu) ☐ ☐ ☐ ☐

Beans ☐ ☐

Water ☐ ☐ ☐ ☐ ☐ ☐ ☐ ☐

Tranquility Break

Be here, now. Practice mindfulness: Notice the colors, textures, sounds, and scents around you— no matter what you're doing.

Splurges, extras, and oversize portions: _____

_____

_____

Best food choice today: _____

_____

_____

Exercise Log

Walking or other aerobic activity: _____ minutes

Strength training: Upper body ☐   Lower body ☐   Core ☐

My "lifestyle activity" choices included: _____

_____

_____

Stress-Soothing Check-In

My stress level today: Low ☐   Medium ☐   High ☐   Red Alert ☐

I reduced my stress by: _____

_____

_____

My thoughts and feelings about my food, exercise, and stress-relief choices today:

_____

_____

_____

_____

_____

_____

_____

_____

_____

_____

_____

_____

_____

_____

_____

_____

_____

_____

_____

_____

_____

_____

_____

GET YOURSELF MOVING!

Twice a day, walk your dog for 15 minutes. You'll get in a 30-minute walk—and so will your pooch.

Check off each serving you eat of these *Sugar Solution* superfoods:

Fruit ☐ ☐ ☐ ☐

Vegetables ☐ ☐ ☐ ☐

Whole grains ☐ ☐ ☐ ☐ ☐ ☐ ☐ ☐

Low-fat or fat-free dairy products ☐ ☐ ☐

Good fats (in half-servings) ☑ ☑ ☑

Nuts (in half-servings) ☑

Lean protein (including eggs, lean meats, poultry, and tofu) ☐ ☐ ☐ ☐

Beans ☐ ☐

Water ☐ ☐ ☐ ☐ ☐ ☐ ☐ ☐

Tranquility Break

Say om. Meditation can decrease circular, ruminative thinking— those times when you chew on the same downbeat thoughts over and over again.

Splurges, extras, and oversize portions: _____
_____
_____

Best food choice today: _____
_____
_____

Exercise Log

Walking or other aerobic activity: _____ minutes

Strength training: Upper body ☐   Lower body ☐   Core ☐

My "lifestyle activity" choices included: _____
_____
_____

Stress-Soothing Check-In

My stress level today: Low ☐   Medium ☐   High ☐   Red Alert ☐

I reduced my stress by: _____
_____
_____

My thoughts and feelings about my food, exercise, and stress-relief choices today:

_____

_____

_____

_____

_____

_____

_____

_____

_____

_____

_____

_____

_____

_____

_____

_____

_____

_____

_____

_____

_____

GET YOURSELF MOVING!

When you go to the supermarket, carry a basket instead of pushing a cart. It's an easy way to challenge your muscles.

Check off each serving you eat of these *Sugar Solution* superfoods:

Fruit ☐ ☐ ☐ ☐

Vegetables ☐ ☐ ☐ ☐

Whole grains ☐ ☐ ☐ ☐ ☐ ☐ ☐ ☐

Low-fat or fat-free dairy products ☐ ☐ ☐

Good fats (in half-servings) ☑ ☑ ☑

Nuts (in half-servings) ☑

Lean protein (including eggs, lean meats, poultry, and tofu) ☐ ☐ ☐ ☐

Beans ☐ ☐

Water ☐ ☐ ☐ ☐ ☐ ☐ ☐ ☐

Tranquility Break

Whine (within limits). Call a friend, and tell her that you're stressed and just need 2 minutes or so to unload. Her job is to listen without interrupting. When you're done, reciprocate.

Splurges, extras, and oversize portions: _____

_____

_____

Best food choice today: _____

_____

_____

Exercise Log

Walking or other aerobic activity: _____ minutes

Strength training: Upper body ☐   Lower body ☐   Core ☐

My "lifestyle activity" choices included: _____

_____

_____

Stress-Soothing Check-In

My stress level today: Low ☐   Medium ☐   High ☐   Red Alert ☐

I reduced my stress by: _____

_____

_____

My thoughts and feelings about my food, exercise, and stress-relief choices today:

_____

_____

_____

_____

_____

_____

_____

_____

_____

_____

_____

_____

_____

_____

_____

_____

_____

_____

_____

_____

_____

_____

GET YOURSELF MOVING!

At home or work, get up every hour and move for 5 minutes. Stretch, flex, pace. If you work 8 hours a day, that's 40 minutes of physical activity you wouldn't have otherwise accrued. To help you remember, put a reminder on your computer or set an alarm clock.

Check off each serving you eat of these _Sugar Solution_ superfoods:

Fruit	☐ ☐ ☐ ☐
Vegetables	☐ ☐ ☐ ☐
Whole grains	☐ ☐ ☐ ☐ ☐ ☐ ☐ ☐
Low-fat or fat-free dairy products	☐ ☐ ☐
Good fats (in half-servings)	☑ ☑ ☑
Nuts (in half-servings)	☑
Lean protein (including eggs, lean meats, poultry, and tofu)	☐ ☐ ☐ ☐
Beans	☐ ☐
Water	☐ ☐ ☐ ☐ ☐ ☐ ☐ ☐

Tranquility Break

Splurge on colorful flowers. Research shows that a bright bouquet of posies lowers women's stress better than green foliage-only plants.

Splurges, extras, and oversize portions: _____
_____
_____

Best food choice today: _____
_____
_____

Exercise Log

Walking or other aerobic activity: _____ minutes

Strength training: Upper body ☐   Lower body ☐   Core ☐

My "lifestyle activity" choices included: _____
_____
_____

Stress-Soothing Check-In

My stress level today: Low ☐   Medium ☐   High ☐   Red Alert ☐

I reduced my stress by: _____
_____
_____

My thoughts and feelings about my food, exercise, and stress-relief choices today:

_____

_____

_____

_____

_____

_____

_____

_____

_____

_____

_____

_____

_____

_____

_____

_____

_____

_____

_____

_____

_____

_____

GET YOURSELF MOVING!

Instead of sitting in your car at the drive-up window of the drugstore, bank, or other business, park and walk inside.

Check off each serving you eat of these *Sugar Solution* superfoods:

Fruit ☐ ☐ ☐ ☐

Vegetables ☐ ☐ ☐ ☐

Whole grains ☐ ☐ ☐ ☐ ☐ ☐ ☐ ☐

Low-fat or fat-free dairy products ☐ ☐ ☐

Good fats (in half-servings) ☑ ☑ ☑

Nuts (in half-servings) ☑

Lean protein (including eggs, lean meats, poultry, and tofu) ☐ ☐ ☐ ☐

Beans ☐ ☐

Water ☐ ☐ ☐ ☐ ☐ ☐ ☐

Tranquility Break

Target your clutter zones. Disorganization makes you feel out of control. Choose one of your home's crazy spots, and spend 10 minutes chucking what you don't need and putting the rest where it belongs.

Splurges, extras, and oversize portions: _____
_____
_____

Best food choice today: _____
_____
_____

Exercise Log

Walking or other aerobic activity: _____ minutes

Strength training: Upper body ☐   Lower body ☐   Core ☐

My "lifestyle activity" choices included: _____
_____
_____

Stress-Soothing Check-In

My stress level today: Low ☐   Medium ☐   High ☐   Red Alert ☐

I reduced my stress by: _____
_____
_____

My thoughts and feelings about my food, exercise, and stress-relief choices today:

_____

_____

_____

_____

_____

_____

_____

_____

_____

_____

_____

_____

_____

_____

_____

_____

_____

_____

_____

_____

GET YOURSELF MOVING!

Tell yourself that taking a walk will help you accomplish more on your to-do list. Exercise makes you feel better and think more clearly, so you become more productive.

WEEK 4 REVIEW

DATE _____ DAY_____

My weight at the end of the week: _____ **Weight change this week:** _____

My biggest successes and choices I'm most proud of regarding . . .

Diet: _____

_____

Exercise: _____

_____

Stress reduction: _____

_____

Biggest challenges this week—and how I met them—regarding . . .

Diet: _____

_____

Exercise: _____

_____

Stress reduction: _____

_____

Lessons I learned this week:

_____

_____

_____

_____

Patterns I noticed this week related to eating, exercise, or stress:

_____

_____

_____

_____

SIX BLOOD SUGAR LOWERING SECRETS

When it comes to getting more "good" carbs in your diet to keep blood sugar levels on even keel, here are six things to remember.

1. **Include one per meal.** Try to choose one-third to one-half of your daily starches from our list of foods low on the glycemic index (GI) (see page 66), a system that ranks carbohydrates based on how high they raise your blood sugar. You're well on your way if you include one low-GI starch—for instance, a bowl of old-fashioned oatmeal, $^1/_2$ cup beans, or some lentil soup—per meal.

2. **Go whole grain.** There are exceptions, but in general, whole grain–based foods such as barley and bulgur have low GIs, mainly because their high fiber content slows digestion.

3. **Rough it up.** The less processed and the rougher the grain or flour, the lower its GI. That's why pasta, which is made from a coarse-milled wheat, has a low GI, even though it's not whole grain.

4. **Bring it down low.** Only have time to make instant rice? Just add some beans. Throwing in a low-GI food brings down the GI rating of the entire meal. Adding some fat or protein also lowers the GI level.

5. **Be savvy about snacks.** When you snack, you tend to have just one food, all by itself. That's fine if you're having a low-cal snack, whether the GI is high or not. But if you're having a high-GI bagel or doughnut with hundreds of calories, the glucose won't get blunted by other foods. So avoid starchy, high-GI foods as snacks.

6. **Load up on fruits, vegetables, and legumes.** Most have a low GI, and you'd have to eat pounds of even those with a high GI to affect blood sugar. But by the same token, don't binge on low-GI foods that are high in calories, such as Snickers candy bars. Gaining weight will raise your blood sugar, too.

LOW-GLYCEMIC CARBS

These foods all have a glycemic-index (GI) ranking below 55, qualifying them as "low GI." The lower the number, the less impact the food will have on your blood sugar. Note: Portions and calories still count! Eat low-GI foods in the controlled serving sizes recommended by the *Sugar Solution* plan. (For more portion info, see pages vii and 73.)

Artichoke	<15	Apple	36
Asparagus	<15	Pear	36
Broccoli	<15	Whole wheat spaghetti	37
Cauliflower	<15	Tomato soup	38
Celery	<15	Carrots, cooked	39
Cucumber	<15	Apple juice	41
Eggplant	<15	Spaghetti	41
Green beans	<15	All-Bran	42
Lettuce, all varieties	<15	Canned chickpeas	42
Low-fat yogurt, artificially sweetened	<15	Grapes	43
Peanuts	<15	Orange	43
Peppers, all varieties	<15	Canned lentil soup	44
Snow peas	<15	Canned pinto beans	45
Spinach	<15	Macaroni	45
Young summer squash	<15	Pineapple juice	46
Zucchini	<15	Long-grain rice	47
Tomatoes	15	Parboiled rice	47
Cherries	22	Bulgur	48
Peas, dried	22	Canned baked beans	48
Plum	24	Grapefruit juice	48
Grapefruit	25	Green peas	48
Pearl barley	25	Oat-bran bread	48
Peach	28	Old-fashioned oatmeal	49
Canned peaches, natural juice	30	Cheese tortellini	50
Dried apricots	31	Canned kidney beans	52
Soy milk	30	Kiwifruit	52
Baby lima beans, frozen	32	Orange juice, not from concentrate	52
Fat-free milk	32	Banana	53
Fettuccine	32	Special K	54
		Sweet potato	54

PLANNER FOOD CHOICES

Choosing foods that are lower on the glycemic index (GI) for breakfast, lunch, dinner, and snacks can help keep your blood sugar lower and steadier all day. Research shows that the more low-GI foods you eat, the better your blood sugar control—but even swapping out one high-GI item for a lower-GI food choice can have a significant impact on your blood sugar, experts say. These suggestions can help.

BREAKFAST

Eat This	Instead of This
Tomato juice	Orange juice
Apple juice	Cranberry juice cocktail
Grapefruit	Cantaloupe
Peach	Raisins
Bran Buds	Rice Krispies
Old-fashioned oatmeal	Quick-cooking oatmeal
All-Bran	Corn flakes
Muesli	Cheerios
Multigrain hot cereal	Instant Cream of Wheat
Sourdough toast	Plain bagel
Pumpernickel toast	English muffin
Stone-ground whole wheat toast	White toast
Oatmeal buttermilk pancakes	Waffles
Raisin bran	Puffed wheat
Strawberries	Strawberry jam

LUNCH

Eat This	Instead of This
Minestrone soup	Chicken with rice soup
Sandwich on whole wheat pita	Sandwich on kaiser roll
Peanut butter and fruit spread on whole wheat bread	PB&J on white bread
Macaroni salad	Potato salad
Three-bean salad	Carrot-raisin salad
Apple	Cookie
Tomato soup	Pea soup
Low-fat sweetened yogurt	Low-fat artificially sweetened yogurt

SNACKS

Eat This	Instead of This
Peanuts	Pretzels
Popcorn	Corn chips
Blueberry muffin	Scone
Pound cake	Angel food cake
Ryvita Crispbread	Rice crackers
Stoned Wheat Thins	Rice cakes
Saltines	Wasa bread crackers
Pear	Pineapple
Plums	Mango
Orange	Candy
Strawberries	Instant pudding

DINNER

Eat This	Instead of This
Converted rice	Instant rice
Brown rice	Couscous (from refined wheat flour)
Long-grain white rice	Instant rice
Boiled new potato	Baked potato
Sweet potato	Instant mashed potatoes
Yams	French fries
Spaghetti cooked al dente	White rice
Pearl barley	Bread stuffing
Sourdough roll	Hamburger bun
Ravioli with meat	Macaroni and cheese
Lentils or lima beans	Bread stuffing
Baked beans or kidney beans	Kaiser roll
Whole wheat spaghetti	Macaroni
Broccoli (second helping)	White bread, white rice, or pasta
Baked beans	Hot dog roll

16 BLOOD SUGAR FRIENDLY SUPERFOODS

Try to fit some of these smart foods into your diet every day. Each has special powers—protein, fiber, good fats, and/or a wealth of nutrients—that keep blood sugar lower and steadier and help protect your body against metabolic changes that lead to insulin resistance (when cells ignore insulin's signal to absorb blood sugar). Insulin resistance makes weight loss more difficult and raises your risk for diabetes, heart disease, and even infertility, memory problems, and some forms of cancer. The health benefits can't be beat . . . but best of all, these superfoods simply taste great!

ALMONDS

1 serving: ½ ounce (11 to 12 almonds); 90 calories

Packed with monounsaturated fat, protein, and fiber, almonds can help keep blood sugar lower and steadier by slowing the absorption of glucose from carbohydrate-rich foods into your bloodstream after you eat. Toss into salads, stir-fries, fruit salad, and hot or cold cereal.

APPLES

1 serving: 1 medium; 80 calories

Apples are a rich source of pectin, a soluble fiber that slows the digestion of carbohydrates (such as fruits, veggies, and grains). For a portable snack, slice an apple and place in a zip-plastic bag with 2 teaspoons of cinnamon. It tastes like apple pie, minus crust and sugar.

AVOCADO

1 serving: ¼–½ of an avocado; about 150 calories

Full of "good" monounsaturated fats that fight the inflammation that can lead to insulin resistance, avocados are best used as a replacement for other high-fat stuff such as cheese or butter, which are rich in saturated fats that researchers suspect contribute to insulin resistance.

BERRIES

1 serving: ½ cup; about 60 calories

Bursting with flavor, full of fiber, and loaded with superhealthy antioxidants, berries—from wild blueberries and cranberries to strawberries, raspberries, and blackberries—are a low-glycemic treat you deserve to enjoy year-round. Keep frozen berries on hand for a healthier frozen dessert: Whirl with fat-free milk and sugar substitute in a food processor.

BROCCOLI

Serving size: 1 medium stalk; 50 calories

The powerful glucoraphanin in broccoli boosts the body's entire antioxidant defense system so that it can disarm lots of free radicals and cool inflammation that may trigger insulin resistance. Sprinkle finely chopped broccoli florets over casseroles, soups, and salads.

CINNAMON

1 serving: ½ teaspoon; 0 calories

This pungent spice makes muscle and liver cells more sensitive to the hormone insulin, reducing insulin resistance and keeping blood sugar lower. Sprinkle a little on your morning coffee or cocoa or use in place of salt and pepper on baked sweet potatoes.

KIDNEY BEANS

1 serving: ½ cup; 112 calories

Soluble fiber and protein in these yummy beans regulate the absorption of glucose into your bloodstream. Rinse canned kidney beans first to remove sodium. Toss 'em into chili, casseroles, and soups.

LEAN BEEF

1 serving: 4 ounces; 240 calories

The protein in beef helps control the way your body handles carbohydrates, slowing digestion so that your blood sugar stays lower and steadier after a meal. Look for the words "lean" or "extra-lean" on the label; these cuts have 4.5 grams or less of saturated fat and 5 to 10 grams of total fat per serving. Or, look for these lean cuts: bottom, eye or top round, round tip, top sirloin, top loin, or tenderloin.

MILK

1 serving: 8 ounces; 110 calories for 1 percent milk, 90 calories for fat-free

Your heart—and your waistline—loves a milk mustache. (So, of course, do your bones!) A growing stack of research proves that calcium and other minerals in milk protect you from insulin resistance and may even help your body burn more fat. Mix 1 cup of fat-free or low-fat milk, two packets of sugar substitute, and 2 to 3 teaspoons of unsweetened cocoa powder in a small saucepan or microwaveable cup. Heat for about 1 minute.

OATMEAL

1 serving: 1–1½ cups, cooked; 145–210 calories

Beta-glucan, the soluble fiber found in oats, acts like a sponge in your intestines—it slows the digestion of carbohydrates and the release of glucose into your bloodstream. Skip the instant stuff: Buy old-fashioned oats, add to boiling water, stir, and turn off the heat. Go take a shower. In 10 minutes, breakfast's ready. Add fruit, nuts, and milk.

SALMON

Serving size: 3–4 ounces (about the size of your palm); about 230 calories

Among omega-3-rich fatty fish, salmon is king: One serving contains about 1.8 grams of eicosapentaenoic acid (EPA) and docosahexaenoic acid (DHA), important omega-3s that cool inflammation. Easy way to get more into your diet: Go for canned salmon. While wild salmon fillets and steaks are difficult to find in most supermarkets (and may cost as much as $28 per pound), canned salmon is a brilliant alternative that usually costs less than $5 per can. Use it in place of tuna to make salmon salad.

SPINACH

1 serving: 1 cup raw, 6 calories; ½ cup cooked, 40 calories

Spinach brims with folate and potassium, heart-healthy nutrients that may also protect against the ravages of prediabetic metabolic syndrome. No time to painstakingly rinse and de-stem each leaf in a bagful of fresh spinach? Grab a microwaveable bag of the prewashed stuff. It's worth the added expense. Slit the bag, add a dab of olive oil and some chopped garlic, then follow the heating directions on the bag.

SWEET POTATOES

1 serving: 1 medium sweet potato; 117 calories

Rated the number one healthiest vegetable by *Nutrition Action Health letter,* the sweet potato is nearly a meal in itself—full of protein, fiber, artery-protecting beta-carotene, blood pressure controlling potassium, and the antioxidant vitamins C and E. Unlike white potatoes, sweet potatoes won't send your blood sugar soaring. Wash and pierce the skin of two sweet potatoes, then microwave on high for 6 to 8 minutes. Mash with a dab of olive oil for a savory tater or with cinnamon for a very sweet treat.

TOMATOES

1 serving: 1 cup sliced tomato, ½ cup sauce, ¾ cup low-sodium tomato juice; 40-60 calories

Whether fresh from the vine, cooked down into a thick sauce, or sun-dried, tomatoes are nutritional wonders. Low on the glycemic index, they're rich in fiber and full-bodied flavor. For tasty, fresh tomatoes when the season's past, try the grape, plum, or on-the-vine types in your supermarket produce department. Give 'em the sniff test: If they smell like ripe tomatoes, chances are they'll taste good, too.

TURKEY

1 serving: 4 ounces; 214 calories

Don't save roast turkey for Thanksgiving. A 4-ounce serving provides 60.3 percent of the hunger-satisfying, blood sugar controlling protein you need in one day, with only half the artery-clogging saturated fat found in most cuts of red meat. Use skinless ground turkey instead of ground beef or ground chicken in recipes for chili, meat loaf, and burgers.

WALNUTS

1 serving: ½ ounce (7 walnut halves); 95 calories

This is the only nut with an appreciable amount of the omega-3 fatty acid called alpha-linolenic acid (ALA), a "good fat" that can help cool off the chronic, bodywide inflammation that may trigger prediabetic changes in the way your cells absorb and burn blood sugar. Carry a snack-size serving in a zip-top bag.

FAST-FOOD GUIDE

We won't tell you to skip the drive-thru; everybody has a busy day now and then, when there's just 10 minutes for lunch or half an hour to get the kids from tuba lessons to soccer practice. Whether you eat on the road or have a few minutes to sit down, the good news is that fast-food choices are healthier than ever—provided you ignore the supersize burgers; fat- and calorie-packed fries; and giant, sugar-laden drinks. We recommend these alternatives.

- **Breakfast:** Choose a plain bagel, toast, or an English muffin rather than a doughnut or muffin, which may be loaded with sugar and fat. Add fruit juice or low-fat or fat-free milk. Also good: cold cereal with fat-free milk, pancakes without butter, or plain scrambled eggs. Limit high-fat bacon, sausage, and cheese, along with the breakfast sandwiches made with them.

- **Lunch and dinner:** Consider a grilled chicken sandwich—regular or junior-size rather than deluxe, and hold the mayo or special sauce. Skip chicken described as "crispy" or "breaded"—it's battered and fried, adding calories and fat. Love burgers? Choose a veggie burger or small hamburger, and hold the cheese. Hold the fries, too. Most fast-food places now have soups and salads. And look for yogurt with fruit and new fruit-and-nut salads. Small orders of chili and baked potatoes topped with veggies are also good choices.

- **Salad bars:** Go for the greens and veggies; use a very light hand with high-fat dressings, bacon bits, cheese, and croutons. Also limit salad bar items like potato or macaroni salad.

- **Mexican fast food:** Stick with bean burritos, soft tacos, fajitas, and other nonfried items; go easy on the cheese, sour cream, and guacamole. Choose chicken over beef, and limit refried beans—but lay on the low-fat, spicy salsa. Pass on anything in a taco shell—a taco salad can pack more than 1,000 calories.

- **Pizza:** Choose thin-crust pizza with vegetable toppings—meat and extra cheese add calories, fat, and sodium—and have only a slice or two.

PORTIONS

Beware of the fattening effects of portion distortion: In one shocking study of real-world foods, New York University nutritionists found that cookies for sale in Manhattan delicatessens were seven times larger than recommended portion sizes, pasta portions served in restaurants were five times larger, and muffins weighed in at triple the size—and calories—of suggested portions. One fast-food chain had relabeled its "medium" fries as "small"—and added even larger portions to the menu. Meanwhile, a University of North Carolina study found that, thanks to bigger portions sold in stores and restaurants, the servings we give ourselves and our families at home are on the rise, too. The result? We may be eating hundreds of calories more each day than we did 20 years ago.

Use these real-world visual cues to keep healthy, calorie-controlled portions in mind, whether you're eating out—or staying home.

FRUIT

1 medium apple or orange = a baseball

½ cup chopped or cooked fruit = an ice-cream scoop or a tennis ball

¼ cup raisins = a mini-muffin wrapper

VEGETABLES

½ cup cooked veggies = a small fist or your palm

1 cup raw vegetables = a large fist

1 medium potato = a computer mouse

GRAINS

½ cup cooked cereal, pasta, or rice = an ice-cream scoop

1 tortilla = a small (7-inch) plate

½ bagel = the width of the lid from a large cup of coffee

1 muffin = a large egg

1 pancake or waffle = a small (4-inch) CD

4 small cookies (like vanilla wafers) = 4 poker chips

1 cup pasta = a tennis ball

Steamed rice = a cupcake wrapper

PROTEIN

3 oz cooked meat, poultry, or fish = a bar of soap

1 oz meat = a matchbox

8 oz meat = a thin paperback

3 oz fish = a checkbook

½ cup beans = an ice-cream scoop

2 Tbsp of peanut butter = a golf ball

1 tsp peanut butter = a large grape

FATS AND OILS

1 tsp margarine or butter = a thumb tip

2 tsp butter = your whole thumb (joint to tip)

1 Tbsp salad dressing = half a golf ball

DAIRY

1 oz of low-fat cheese = an ice cube

1½ oz cheese = 6 dice

2 oz low-fat cheese = 2 dominoes

½ cup of ice cream = half a baseball

SNACKS

1 oz pretzels = a large handful

1 oz nuts = the amount that fits in your cupped palm

A HANDY GUIDE

How to use your hand to track portions:
- Your fist is about the same size as 1 cup of fruit.
- Your thumb (tip to base) is the size of 1 ounce of meat or cheese.
- Your palm (minus fingers) equals 3 ounces of meat, fish, or poultry.
- Your cupped hand equals 1 to 2 ounces of nuts or pretzels.

NINE WORKOUT PROBLEMS—SOLVED

No time? Too tired? Just can't get started? We've pulled together nine top workout obstacles and tried-and-true expert solutions. Read on—then tie up those sneakers and get out there!

Problem: You're a breastfeeding mom.
Solution: Get moderate exercise.

If you've heard that working out affects the quality of your breast milk, here's some advice from researchers: Get out your running shoes, but keep your pace moderate. University of North Carolina at Greensboro (UNCG) researchers found no drop in fatty acids in the breast milk of 14 healthy women after they walked at a moderate pace for 30 minutes. In fact, the concentration of healthy polyunsaturated fats increased.

Moderate exercise might even help pack more nutrients into breast milk by increasing their concentration in the blood, says Cheryl Lovelady, PhD, coauthor of the study and a professor of nutrition at UNCG.

Don't go overboard, though. Intense exercise could deplete energy stores, ratcheting down milk production, says Lovelady. Also, a previous study showed that a vigorous workout may lower the level of an immune-boosting protein in women's breast milk. So keep it moderate—but keep doing it. Aim to get 30 to 45 minutes of exercise (i.e., a brisk walk) most days of the week.

Problem: You're not a morning person.
Solution: Start your routine in bed.

Everyone dreads those dark winter mornings when you wake up so zonked that even hitting the snooze button takes too much energy. "Because your core temperature is at its lowest, physical performance is worst in the morning, especially when it's cold," says Michael Deschenes, PhD, a professor of kinesiology at the College of William and Mary. "When your muscles are cool, they don't generate as much force and are more susceptible to strain and injury."

Whether you're a committed early exerciser or not, it's worth it to get up and get moving because it will make mornings easier. "As your core temperature rises, hormones and endorphins are released, making your limbs feel looser and improving your mood," says Deschenes. These two moves, which emphasize light stretching and toning, are ideal for mornings when you feel groggy.

- **Upper-Body Fan: Warms the torso and facilitates breathing by opening shoulders and upper chest**

    While lying on your back with arms outstretched to the sides and palms up, bring your knees up and roll them to the right side. Turn your head to the left. Try to keep both shoulders touching the bed. Sweep your left palm in a 180-degree arc over your chest to touch your right palm, letting your head follow your arm, then slowly reverse the move. Repeat 10 times, then switch sides.

- **Gentle Crunch: Warms and tones the core**

    Remove the pillow and lie faceup. Bend your knees and plant your feet on the bed. Press your palms into the mattress near your hips. Tighten your abs and lift both shoulder blades off bed. Hold for a complete breath, then lower. Repeat 10 to 15 times. (If your mattress is soft, do this move on the floor.)

Problem: You're so tired, you can't finish your workout.
Solution: Pretend there are springs on your feet.

If you dream it, you can do it. Seriously. Research suggests that our bodies can't distinguish between something we've drummed up in our minds and something we've really done.

When subjects are wired with electrodes and asked to imagine that they're running a race, muscles contract in much the same way they would if the people were actually moving, finds researcher JoAnn Dahlkoetter, PhD, a sports psychologist at Stanford University. (If you've ever felt winded after waking from a chase sequence in your dreams, this makes sense to you.) The way to make this phenomenon work to your advantage? Positive imagery.

"I remember training a woman at the track who was so tired she could hardly move," Dahlkoetter recalls. "When I asked her what sort of pictures popped into her head when she was working out, she admitted to thinking of herself as a fat slug." Dahlkoetter asked the woman to instead imagine that she had springs on her feet or helium balloons lifting her forward. "Changing her thought process changed her whole workout experience; suddenly, she felt light on her feet and able to move faster," Dahlkoetter notes. "She was energized by her workout."

If you're not into spring or balloon fantasies, pretend that the walker or runner a few paces ahead of you has a powerful magnet on her back that's pulling you along. "Once you catch up, take the magnet and put it on the back of the next person in front of you," Dahlkoetter says. "When no one is ahead of you anymore, envision the magnet at the finish line, effortlessly drawing you toward victory."

Problem: You have no time this week.
Solution: Aim for one workout.

Many people say they would like to work out regularly and get in shape—but that they just don't have the time. Virgil Aponte, a personal trainer and owner of the GivStrength Personal Training Web site, suggests those folks start with a commitment to work out just once a week. While one workout a week may not be optimal, it is a whole lot better than no times per week, and it gives you a great platform to launch a more frequent schedule sometime down the road.

Problem: You have no time, ever.
Solution: Plan on paper.

You're busy. We know. But you may have more time for fitness than you think: Americans have twice as much leisure time as we believe we do, found a 2004 Harris Interactive survey of more than 1,550 people. "We average 35 to 40 hours a week of free time," says Geoffrey Godbey, PhD, a professor of leisure studies at Pennsylvania State University. "The catch is that the time comes in small chunks."

To truly take advantage of those bursts of time, set—and write down—superspecific workout goals. "About 90 percent of the research out there has shown again and again that goal setting has a very positive effect by increasing motivation and persistence," says Aimee C. Kimball, PhD, director of mental training at the University of Pittsburgh Medical Center for Sports Medicine.

To help get you on your way, Kimball suggests keeping an exercise journal in which you record your long-term objectives ("I want to complete a marathon") and your daily targets ("I want to walk 5 miles today"). "Every night, write your detailed game plan for the following day, and make sure you've taken into account any obstacles that may come up," Kimball says. Thinking ahead about potential roadblocks is the best way to sidestep them: You'll know when to squeeze in your walk if that late night at the office sneaks up on you.

Finally, at the end of each week, note the problems you encountered, how you dealt with them, and what you've accomplished. That should inspire you to carve out more time for fitness.

Problem: You're not improving.
Solution: Cue the video.

Watching home movies from last Christmas won't help you reach your fitness goals, but tuning in to another kind of video may do just that. "Seeing an image of proper form—a swim stroke, a tennis serve—has been shown to help the brain improve on what the body can do," Dahlkoetter says. As you watch, you imagine you're performing the action you see. All the while, electrical impulses travel from your brain to your muscles, helping your body remember how to perform properly.

Researchers from the University of Liverpool in England discovered that viewing a video of your own athletic feat improves performance by 29 percent, compared with an 8 percent change in a control group. According to Dahlkoetter, the same will happen if you watch highly skilled athletes compete. *Chariots of Fire,* anyone?

Problem: You see workouts as a chore.
Solution: Enlist a buddy.

As soon as you call an activity an obligation, the fun gets sucked out of it. "To turn your workout into something you look forward to, make it your social time, too," says Jan Griscom, a certified personal trainer in New York City and former advisory board member of the American Council on Exercise. The easiest way to do that is to sweat with a pal.

University of Southern California researchers found that working out with a friend is the best predictor of exercise satisfaction. Another study revealed that when you train with someone you care about, you're more likely to stick with your fitness plan so as not to disappoint your partner. Researchers at Indiana University followed 46 couples; some signed up for the gym together, while some joined solo. After a year, the pairs who did it as a team had a mere 6 percent dropout rate, versus 43 percent for those who opted to go it alone.

Problem: You're too distracted to focus on working out.
Solution: Invest in an iPod.

"Listening to music shuts down the analytical side of the brain," Kimball says. "When you're engrossed in music, your mind can't tell you that you're tired or in pain or should be doing something else." A recent study of 41 overweight women who participated in a 24-week diet-and-walking program found that those who listened to tunes of their choice lost twice as much weight as a group moving without a sound track.

"The music functions as a positive distraction, making you feel like you're not exercising as hard, so the women were able to do the workout more easily," says study author Christopher A. Capuano, PhD, an associate professor of psychology at Fairleigh Dickinson University in Teaneck, New Jersey.

Problem: Your enthusiasm is MIA.
Solution: Love your reflection.

The mirror is a tricky thing. Your reflection can be either friend or foe, depending on your mood. But if you normally find your image pleasing, especially while flexing your muscles, working out in full view of yourself may give you a mental boost, says Jeffrey A. Katula, PhD, a researcher at Wake Forest University in Winston-Salem, North Carolina, who recently published a small study regarding the benefits of exercising in front of a mirror. He reported that if you feel good—pleased that you got yourself to the gym and that you're trying to improve yourself—then "the mirror can reinforce those positive feelings and potentially spur you to do more."

Give your mirror even more positive power by sticking a Post-it note on it that reads something like "I'm getting stronger every day," suggests Steven Ungerleider, PhD, a sports psychologist and author of *Mental Training for Peak Performance.* "A constant encouraging reminder can help motivate you," he says.

CALORIE-BURN CHARTS

How many calories will you burn cooking dinner, walking for an hour, or taking care of a child? You'll find the answers here. The calories are for an hour of activity for a 150-pound person. If your current weight is closer to 175 pounds, add about 15 percent; if you weigh 200 pounds, add about 20 percent. Over 200 pounds? Add about 30 percent.

EVERYDAY ACTIVITIES

Eating	85
Knitting	85
Reading	90
Sewing	85
Shopping	180
Shoveling snow	430
Sitting (watching TV)	70
Sitting (writing, typing)	105
Sleeping	55
Standing	100

DANCING

Aerobic, ballet or fast modern dance	422
Ballroom dancing, fast	387
Ballroom dancing, slow	211
Belly dancing	300–550
Social dance	317

PLAYING AN INSTRUMENT

Playing a cello, flute, horn, or woodwind	141
Playing drums	281
Playing guitar in a band	211
Playing guitar while sitting down	141
Playing a keyboard, violin, or trumpet	176

EXERCISE

Aerobics	450
Aikido	700
Bicycling (5.5 mph)	450
Bicycling (10 mph)	700
Boxing, in the ring	850
Boxing, using a punching bag	422
Elliptical trainer (intense)	700
Elliptical trainer (moderate)	300
Jogging (5 mph)	500
Jump rope (70 jumps per minute)	700
Jump rope (125 jumps per minute)	850
Kickboxing	400
Pilates (intense)	400
Pilates (light)	200
Pilates (moderate)	300
Power walking	600
Rowing (intense)	700
Rowing (moderate)	550
Running (10-minute-mile pace)	850
Running (11:30-minute-mile pace)	700
Stairclimbing (intense)	700
Stairclimbing (moderate)	430
Step aerobics	550
Swimming (vigorous)	500
Tae bo (intense)	800
Tae bo (moderate)	500
Tae kwon do (intense)	700
Tai chi (moderate)	400
Walking (3 mph)	450
Walking (4.5–5 mph)	700
Water aerobics (intense)	700

Water aerobics (moderate) 400

Weight lifting (intense)... 430

Weight lifting (moderate) 215

Yoga 400–600

HOUSEHOLD CHORES AND REPAIRS

Automobile repair 211

Carpentry, general 246

Carrying heavy loads, such as bricks 563

Childcare: sitting/kneeling—dressing, feeding 211

Childcare: standing—dressing, feeding 246

Cleaning, heavy 317

Cleaning, light.. 176

Cleaning, moderate.. 246

Construction, outside, remodeling 387

Cooking, food preparation.. 176

Electrical work, plumbing 246

Moving household furniture.. 422

Painting, papering, plastering, scraping 281

Pushing or pulling stroller with child 176

Scrubbing floors on hands and knees 387

Sweeping garage or sidewalk 281

Vacuuming 180

Window washing 180

YARD WORK

Bagging leaves 322

Chopping wood 486

Clearing land.. 404

Digging, spading, tilling 404

Double digging a garden 688

Gardening with heavy powertools 486

General gardening 404

YARD WORK (CONT.)

Laying sod 404

Mowing lawn (push mower) 486

Mowing lawn (push mower with motor) 364

Mowing lawn (riding) 202

Planting seedlings 324

Planting trees 364

Raking 322

Shoveling heavy snow 728

Shoveling snow 486

Snow thrower (walking) 364

Trimming shrubs (manual) 364

Trimming shrubs (power) 284

Watering lawn or garden 122

Weeding 364

RECREATIONAL ACTIVITIES AND SPORTS

Backpacking 493

Badminton, competitive 493

Badminton, social 317

Basketball, coaching 493

Basketball, competitive 563

Basketball, pick-up game 422

Basketball, shooting baskets 317

Basketball, wheelchair 457

Bicycling, BMX or mountain biking 598

Billiards 176

Bowling 211

Canoeing, light effort 281

Croquet 176

Darts, wall or lawn 176

Diving, springboard or platform 211

RECREATIONAL ACTIVITIES AND SPORTS (CONT.)

Skiing, cross-country, moderate effort 563

Skiing, cross-country, vigorous effort 633

Skiing, downhill, light effort 352

Skiing, downhill, moderate effort 422

Skiing, downhill racing 563

Skiing, water 422

Skimobiling, water 493

Sledding, tobogganing, bobsledding, luge 493

Snorkeling 352

Snowmobiling 246

Snowshoeing 563

Soccer, casual 493

Soccer, competitive 704

Softball, coaching 422

Softball or baseball, fast or slow pitch 352

Squash 844

Surfing, body or board 211

Swimming, leisurely 422

Table tennis 281

Unicycling 563

Volleyball, beach 563

Volleyball, competitive 281

Volleyball, noncompetitive 211

Volleyball, water 211

Water polo 704

Whitewater rafting, kayaking, or canoeing 352

DE-STRESS FOR LOWER BLOOD SUGAR

The ultimate mind-body connection: Lower your stress and you'll not only feel like you've spent an afternoon being pampered at a spa, you'll be taking the first steps toward lowering your blood sugar. In a landmark Duke University study, researchers found that people with diabetes who learned simple mindfulness meditation techniques got lower, healthier readings on a gold-standard test of long-term blood sugar.

You can, too, with these easy stress-reducing techniques.

Relax with a 3-Minute Meditation

Find a quiet space that's both private and inspiring. It can be outside, in a church or temple—even a corner of your bedroom. Sit or lie down, close your eyes (to help you relax), and set a kitchen timer for 3 minutes, so there's no need to worry about when to end the meditation. As your comfort level rises, gradually increase the length of time you meditate to 20 minutes a day.

1. **Be still.**

2. **Invite in the divine.** Make your meditation space a sanctuary for spiritual practice by adding an element or two from your spiritual life—perhaps a candle, crystals, a cross, a Buddha, a picture of your understanding of God, even a tiny bunch of flowers—to remind you of why you're there.

3. **Have a spiritual intention.** Start by repeating an affirming mantra, one that's spiritual and meaningful to you. Use it to help empty your mind and to relax as fully as you can. Then visualize what it is that you want out of life—what you want your world to include and how you want it to feel. Next, actually invoke the presence of the divine, thanking God or the universe for what you have—or simply asking for help in the meditation process.

4. **Pay attention to what comes up.** In the stillness you create, you will notice thoughts or feelings—some of them negative, some of them not—that you may not have been aware of because you had been masking them with activity. Don't try to make them go away. They are what's truly in your heart.

5. **Surrender.** In other words, accept that things don't always go according to your plan. Relax under the strain of your self-imposed rules and actions. Dispense with your frustration or any negative emotions you might feel. Trust that everything will be okay. And surrender to the idea that miracles are your highest potential.

De-Stress with Circle Breathing

Whenever you feel stressed, remember that you have a choice: to practice stress or to practice peace. Then take 5 or 10 circle breaths. Soon your body and mind will shift into circle breathing automatically when you're scattered, anxious, or off center. Make it your goal to try this centering exercise 10 times a day this week, if possible. That will help your body and mind form a strong, positive habit.

1. Inhale and stretch your arms over your head, giving a sigh of relief and lowering your arms as you exhale. Relax and keep your arms lowered for the rest of the exercise.

2. Now imagine that you're inhaling a stream of peaceful energy into a spot a few inches below your navel.

3. Inhale the warm stream into the base of your spine, then imagine it traveling up your back to the top of your head.

4. Exhale and mentally follow your out breath back down the front of your body to the point below the navel where you'll begin the next in breath. Your breath has now made a full circle: up the back of your body, down the front, and back to the starting place below your navel.

5. Continue this breathing pattern for 5 to 10 breaths. You can also use circle breathing for a longer period as a relaxing form of meditation.